LENDING LIBRARY

Unity of the Triangle
5570 Munford Rd.
Raleigh, NC 27612

Phone: 919-832-8324
Website: unitytriangle.org

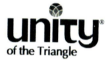

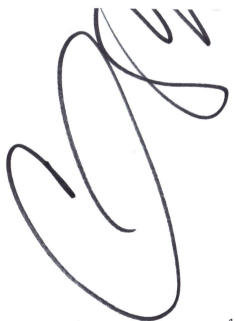

1

This book is dedicated to my family, my best

friends Kiki and Ashley, and the love of my life

Dennis.

Contents

Cherish Yourself

Shana Perkins

Introduction

I believe the goal in everyone's life is simply to be happy. Yet in this world of constant distractions and excessive stimulation, sometimes it's easy to lose track of what's really important and get caught up striving for superficial pleasures. The problem is that after reaching the goals that give you instant gratification it generally doesn't take long for that empty feeling to return, and you have to begin the process of trying to be happy all over again. I think happiness involves finding meaning in all aspects of your life, and the material wants are just here to be icing on the cake, not the cake itself. Too many times I have been caught up in increasing the quantity of stuff in my life without increasing the quality. This has always been a recipe for disaster.

Sick and tired of being sick and tired, I began my search on how to lead a life I could be proud of. Where happiness and success were always felt and not something I had to be constantly working for. Through much study and constant trial and error I found that when you really get down to it, it's the basics that really have the power to shape your life and make you feel good. Happiness comes naturally when you reach a place of satisfaction and comfort in your day-to-day living. Ideally, you want to stay in a state of balance where your mental, physical, and emotional outlets are all in harmony with one another and you enjoy a feeling of inner-peace. I have found when that happens your life just seems to "work" and a lot of the unnecessary stresses we have tend to fall away.

You can choose right now to better yourself and your life, it's not hard. It all starts with a decision. The power of making the decision to elevate your life is greater than any obstacle you will face. The greatest moment in my life was the second I decided I was going to cherish myself. The second greatest was realizing that I am worth it.

Why is it that so many people suffer from inferiority complexes? A lack of self-confidence is probably the biggest hindrance for anyone trying to make gains in their life. When you don't believe you deserve something your subconscious will sabotage any efforts you make. So before you waste any time or energy on making your life better, make sure you know in your heart that you are worth having a better life. Health and happiness are your birthrights, and no matter what mistakes you may have made in the past you deserve nothing but the best.

When is the last time you were cherished? Have you taken time to relax and have fun today? What about yesterday? You should be smiling and enjoying yourself every day! You should feel unbelievable in your own skin and proud of the life that you created for yourself. You are the creator of your own life experience and you set the tone for how you are to be treated by the world by how you treat yourself. Don't you think it's important to start cherishing yourself today?

Cherishing yourself is more than dressing yourself up in fancy clothes or getting the occasional massage. Cherishing yourself is about reaching optimal states of health, happiness, and an overall satisfaction in every area of your life. To be super successful in your career while letting your health fall apart is not success. Neither is becoming overly obsessed with health while letting it interfere in your relationships.

This book will take you through the process of creating balance and joy in all areas, and I hope you enjoy the process of transforming your life into one of abundance. My view of cherishing yourself is to begin with your mental state. All things are created first in the mind, so creating a picture of how you would like for things to be is the first step. Next I want you to have a solid foundation where you do work that fulfills you, enjoy love and support from those you respect and care for, and strengthen those things I call your "Primary Foods". After your foundation is established I want to help you cherish your body through nutrition and give you tools to help you be most effective. Making simple changes in your views and actions will radically transform your life at a profound speed. I congratulate you on making a wonderful decision to bring your wellness to a superior level and wish you the best on your journey.

Note from Shana...

I want to help you cherish yourself so that you feel amazing every day. I want you to get to a place where making the right decisions is effortless. You should feel so good that you get up in the morning with a huge supply of energy ready to tackle the day and the world. Experience the beauty of having goals and aspirations worthy of you and that add excitement and bring hope to your life. Above all I want you to learn to love and appreciate yourself for the magnificent being you are. I also want to supply you with the tools to support you in the ever-evolving process that is life. Give yourself a chance to realize you deserve all the abundance the Universe has to offer and allow yourself to grow and change. It all starts with the vision you have of your life and yourself and as you change your vision you change

your life.

Create your vision

Creating your life is something everyone does every second of every day. Unfortunately, most people don't realize they have the power to do it consciously so they let their subconscious wreak havoc upon their existence. The purpose of this book is to show you that you have had the power all along and how easy it is to use this power to create a life of happiness and abundance. There is a process that I am going to show you and it is all based in fact. Just like the Law of Gravity, there are other laws governing the Universe in which you live, and when you can learn to live in harmony with those laws instead of fighting them (which is always going to be a losing battle) then you will thrive and excel in all areas of your life. There are so many laws in this world, some known and I suspect many others unknown. Throughout these pages I will be giving examples of laws taken from different religions, philosophers, writers, and the great minds throughout history.

Look at everything in your life right now: the home you live in, the relationships you have, your career and your health. All of these things are the result of your past focus and are mirroring yourself back at you. When you learn to redirect your focus, all these things change as if by magic. The Law of Attraction teaches us that like attracts like, basically what we think about is drawn to us. So when you put your attention on the current situation you always end up getting more of the same. This is sometimes hard for people to comprehend. You might be thinking that this can't possibly be true. I didn't attract all this negativity in my life! I never thought about my husband cheating on me, my weight problem or this disease. I hate to break it to you, but even though those particular thoughts might not have crossed your mind I can assure you that you did attract them by thinking thoughts of a similar nature and vibration.

Everything in the universe is essentially energy and has a particular vibration, it basically boils down to things that make you happy have one type of vibration while things that make you unhappy are on a different frequency. That's why things tend to snowball downhill when something happens and you can't get out of your funk. That's also why when people hit rock-bottom they tend to feel better and relax because they know it can't get any worse and they begin attracting things in their life that are on a positive vibration. For in-depth learning on the law of attraction Jerry and Esther Hicks are excellent, and I highly recommend picking up a book by them.

Of course it's not as easy as simply sitting on your couch and dreaming of a new car and expecting one to pull up in your driveway. Life doesn't work like that. Everything worth having in life is worth working for. You don't appreciate what you don't work for anyway. I want to help you by teaching you how to work the right way and saving you from wasting unnecessary time and energy. No one says you have to work hard; you just have to work smart. Make what you do in this life count. It is still uncertain on whether or not you are going to get another chance.

Now that you understand that you are where you are in life because of what you have been focusing on, it's time to get to where you really want to be by redirecting your attention to what you want your future to look like. You have to create a new vision of yourself, but before you can create the person you want to become, you have to accept and embrace the person you are now. We all have habits and struggles we have been trying to overcome, but they are so ingrained with the idea we have of ourselves in our head that it becomes a losing battle. You will find that as you change your identity these habits will fall away much more easily.

Please don't berate yourself for where you are now! This is so important I cannot over emphasize it. Whatever has happened to you in your life it has brought you to this place of wanting to grow and has taught you many lessons along the way that will help you for the rest of your days. Love and appreciate yourself and be thankful for exactly where you are because exactly where you are is going to take you to exactly where you want to end up. Above all, this is a journey you want to enjoy taking because you cannot reach a happy destination without having a happy journey. Every second is precious and you always have the choice whether you are going to move in the direction of where you want to be or if you are going to continue to do what you have always done and stay in the same place. The definition of insanity is doing the same thing over and over and expecting a different result.

Back to your vision of yourself. I want you to imagine yourself as an artist and the new image of yourself that you are about to paint is going to be your masterpiece. Start thinking about exactly the person you want to be. What does this person look like? What are their habits? What do they choose for a career? Does this person have a life's mission that they want to accomplish or do they simply want to relax and enjoy the beauty of each day? Whatever you choose for yourself is the right answer. As long as your choices do not hurt another, there is no limit and no wrong answers. Whatever the mind can conceive and believe... the mind can achieve.

Now that you have a crystal clear vision of your ideal version of yourself, it's time to start acting as if you know for a fact that this person is coming. You are in the process of a great transformation and can relax because you are about to be exactly who you want to be. You are a caterpillar about to turn into a beautiful butterfly. Don't worry about how you are going to do it right now, just relax and be confident and secure in your knowledge that it IS coming.

Each moment you spend thinking of yourself being and having exactly what you want, and you do it in a spirit of joy and happiness, you are bringing this version closer to you. When your belief starts to crystallize into absolute faith, the speed in which it is delivered is quickened. As you proceed with your visualization you will start to get feedback from the Universe by having flashes of inspiration come into your mind. Follow these hunches! These are the necessary actions to take for you to make the change into who you want to become. Your life is like your own private movie and you are the director. The Universe doesn't care what your script is; it is going to give you exactly what you want. How you communicate and tell it what you want is by the thoughts you choose to think. That is why you have what you have, by thinking what you have been thinking.

Napoleon Hill spent 20 years studying the laws of success and he discovered that everything begins in the mind. It all starts with having a definite purpose in life. Feeding that purpose, thoughts laced with desire and excitement until it becomes a burning obsession is critical for achieving any goal whether it be money, fame, health or all of the above. He also found that all people who succeed are met with some temporary setbacks and failures and usually success was met shortly after for the few who chose to keep on fighting. The Universe or Infinite Intelligence as it also called, works in mysterious ways and your obstacles are really just opportunities in disguise. Keep in mind that every adversity has the seed of an equivalent or greater benefit and you will find it much easier to approach your obstacles with the right attitude.

Keeping the right attitude is critical because you are ALWAYS attracting things into your life and you want to make sure that you are attracting things that are on the right vibration. You don't get to choose when you want to start attracting and because of that it are necessary to pay attention to your emotions. Paying attention to your emotions is the easiest way to know if you are bringing the things you want closer to your life or not. It's really very simple; when you feel good you are attracting more things in which to feel good about and when you feel bad you are attracting more things that will make you feel bad.

The emotions you feel are largely a result of your inner dialogue. Everyone has a voice in their head that has a comment on everything. The sad thing is that most people's voices are constantly putting themselves down. Pay attention to your voice from now on. Is it making you feel badly by focusing on your flaws? When you look in the mirror are your eyes going to all the spots you think are less than perfect? Can you accept a compliment fully and completely without saying that you could have done something better? When you can turn that voice in your head into your biggest cheerleader you will make drastic progress.

Wouldn't it be nice to have constant support and encouragement? Most people wouldn't dream of talking to their friends or loved ones the way they talk to themselves. Be your best friend and start the best habit you can, which is to NEVER put yourself down. Instead start thinking about all the things you appreciate and admire about yourself. Having self-respect is the most attractive quality a person can have, and you really can't expect others to respect you if you don't respect yourself.

So from now on you are keeping this ideal version of yourself in your mind throughout the day, while paying attention to your gut feelings (feedback from the Universe). Throughout your day you are making it your number one priority to feel good, and you do this easily by constantly appreciating yourself and being supportive and understanding of everything about you. You are not here to judge yourself and you should not be influenced by others opinions of you either. After all, people are really more self-focused than anything and if they are looking at something in you that they do not like, it is generally just a reflection of something they do not like about themselves. Besides, now you know that any negativity they are putting out is coming back to them, and they are just attracting more of it in their lives! The Law of Karma is always working as well and whatever you put out comes back to you 3 times over. So instead of being upset for yourself, be sorry for them and happy that you now have the knowledge to attract only that which you want into your life. That alone should make you relax and smile and of course attract more good things.

Start making it a daily habit to find things in yourself and in your life that you appreciate. Make it a priority to spend some time each day in nature. Nature is so healing. Getting fresh air, sunshine, and taking in beautiful scenery helps to cleanse the body, get Vitamin

D, and relax the mind. When the mind is relaxed it is much easier to get communication from the Universe, and you will find that you get your best ideas when you are doing simple things and enjoying yourself. When you take walks, shower, drive, or listen to a good piece of music, these actions will help to put you in the right frame of mind to receive inspiration for the attainment of your goals.

Spend time in nature and connect yourself with Mother Earth. There is energy in the Earth that most people are so out of touch with because they rarely ever walk barefoot in the grass or garden with their hands. Try to make it a point to spend some time each day either sitting on the ground, walking barefoot, gardening or anything else than has your skin touching the earth. You will naturally become more grounded the more you do it. Remember everything you do adds up and it all becomes a part of you. You are creating your ideal version of yourself so make each part count.

Always trust your instincts and you will be aptly rewarded. There are so many things that communicate with you besides what you see and hear. Everything has a vibration and energy and you tune in to them without even being aware you are doing it. Animals and children do this naturally. The more you ground yourself and free yourself from your pre-conceived notions, the more in tune you become and the strength of your instincts will grow. One way to help do this is to meditate. Meditation is learning to quiet your mind and reach a state of inner relaxation and peace you so rarely get in the hustle and bustle world you live in. There are many ways in which to meditate. For me, I find it easiest to play music I love and just walk. It took me years to understand why I had a habit of walking around and around the kitchen table listening to music when I was a child as a form of deep relaxation. Even today I get my best ideas when I simple tune out the world and walk. Whatever you can do that is relaxing and shuts your conscious off for a time is deeply beneficial both mentally and physically. Be prepared for flashes of inspiration to come during this time and not when you are searching, as these will be the ideas that help you most when striving towards your goals.

Now that you have a beautiful image of the self that you are in the process of creating, and you have learned that feeling good and being nice to yourself are the starting points of any endeavor, it is time to set goals for yourself. One reason that people fail to reach the goals that they set is they don't realize the importance of setting goals that move them. If you are not emotionally attached to your goals it is much harder to reach them. Set goals worthy of you, goals that you can see yourself

26

obtaining with a sound plan of action. Having goals that excite you makes any work you are required to expend seem effortless. You need to be filled with such a longing to succeed at getting what you want that any obstacles placed in your path are knocked down with your intense desire. There is no question what road you are going to take if one leads to your desire and one away from it. Every day you are moving closer to reaching your goal and you see yourself reaching it in your mind's eye constantly.

Having big goals is more than having dreams. When a dream changes form and turns into a goal, a sound plan of action is produced. You build confidence because you know that it is only a matter of time before you have what your heart desires, and all action that you have to take is done with excitement and in good spirit. When you reach a state where the work you are doing is

27

as much play as it is work you know you have chosen a worthy goal. When you enjoy your work you have reached a new pinnacle of being successful in life.

Now that you have decided on the person you are choosing to become, you have to learn how to make your changes last. The reason it is so hard to make lasting change is most people don't know what drives us to fall back into our old habits and tendencies. Everything we do in life is to achieve pleasure and avoid pain. We need to learn how to control our motives.

"The secret of success is learning how to use pain and pleasure instead of having pain and pleasure use you. If you do that, you're in control of your life. If you don't, life controls you."   Anthony Robbins

In the book <u>Awaken the Giant Within,</u> Anthony Robbins helps you to understand that emotion and not intellect drive human behavior. Sure you may know you want to lose weight, but short term focus and momentary pleasure of that bar of chocolate overrides your intellect and you eat it anyway. Smoking is another clear example of the trouble people have with making a change stick. You feel you simple need that cigarette to calm down right now and that is more important than the fact that you KNOW it contributes to cancer, heart disease and inflammation throughout the entire body.

So how do we rewire our priorities? The secret to making lasting change is a combination of changing our Neuro-Associations and adding the right leverage. Anthony Robbins was able to travel the world demonstrating that when you do this, change can happen in an instant.

Say one of your goals is to lose weight and be healthier; you need to create enough pain associated with being overweight that you hit your emotional pain

29

threshold and it is no longer an issue. Studies show that people base their decisions more on the avoidance of pain than in the attainment of pleasure. So how do you do that? First you need to sit down and list reasons that emotionally move you. Maybe some of your reasons are being able to see your grandchildren grow up or fit into your clothes. Maybe you want your partner to be more attracted to you. Maybe you visualize the pain of having an illness which is directly affected by your body weight. You need to create massive pain in your mind associated with being overweight by having reasons that move you.

Next you need to link pleasure to losing weight and becoming healthier. You need to find the visualizations that create intense emotions on both the pleasure of losing weight and the pain of keeping the weight on, and you need to replay these images in your mind again and again. Using the Law of Reinforcement to drive these new emotions into your mind you can continually keep your focus on what you want it to be on. By doing this often you can utilize the Law of Recency.

The Law of Recency

Things most recently learned are best remembered, while the things learned some time ago are remembered with more difficulty.

So now you have the vision of yourself that you are moving towards and a new set of tools on how to make this person stick around. Next you want to create rewards for yourself every time you make the right choices so you can reinforce your behavior. Do this after every decision you make that brings you closer to your goals and you will be much more successful. The Law of Effect tells us that "learning will always be much more effective when a feeling of pleasantness, satisfaction or reward accompanies or is the result of the learning process".

You are now equipped with a set of useful tools to make your vision become not only a reality, but a reality that will LAST. Next you want to make sure you are in an optimal state of health because that is going to be the foundation for everything you do in life. Our health affects our energy, our drive, our clarity of thinking and our disposition. How on earth can you concentrate on feeling good and reaching for your dreams if your body is in a constant state of dis-ease?

The foundation for having a healthy life is not as cut and dry as you may think. Many things contribute to your over all well-being and I believe the heart of health lies in what I call your Primary Foods.

Primary Foods

One of the best decisions in my life was deciding to go to The Institute for Integrative Nutrition. Having been in the health industry for years doing personal training, nutrition counseling, and practicing alternative forms of medicine, I was mainly planning to enjoy going over knowledge I already had and getting some more credentials. Thank god I was wrong!

I was so lucky to learn about the importance of Primary Food in life and how big a difference it makes. If your Primary food is out of balance you can be eating an optimal diet and still be less than healthy. Health is the most important thing you have and when you make the decision to protect this precious commodity you are making the best investment you can make. Health affects everything, it doesn't matter what you have if you don't have your health you are poor. The foundation for health resides in 4 important Primary foods: spirituality, relationships, physical activity, and career.

Spirituality

When I talk about spirituality I am not referring to any religion, but more of a philosophy that you take with you on your way through life. When you can refer to a set of ethics and morals that are as much a part of you as your physical body, you find an ease in your daily living. When you set your standards high it reflects in everything that you do, and surprisingly life becomes easier and not harder.

There may come a time when you recognize a higher power in life. Something you cannot see, but you can feel deeply. To be able to tune in to the energy of the world changes your perception on all things. Finding your own special philosophy in life is vitally important and is the biggest blessing you can obtain. Decision making takes on much less difficulty because you have a set of beliefs you can refer to, and a huge amount of stress naturally leaves the body as the result of this new paradigm.

Life comes in cycles and having a personal philosophy that is positive in nature will get you through your darkest moments. One of my favorite teachers, Chris Prentiss, made a huge impact on me when I was shown through his book, <u>Change your thinking, Change your life</u>, that when you look at things not only happening for a reason but for your best benefit, you can start to see the perfection of life. Having inspiration in your daily life is like turning on the music and color in the movie you are making. It enhances the beauty of your masterpiece. You can find inspiration through religion, books, music, and anything that changes your perception. All of these have a spiritual quality, and there is no right or wrong way to finding your own guiding light.

When I first read Change Your Thinking, Change your Life, I was 25 years old and so sick I could barely walk to the bathroom. I went to doctor after doctor and no one could find what was wrong. I finally had to move back in with my mother, and I think we were all sort of preparing for me to die. I had lived a life of extreme excess in my teens and early 20's and though I was a personal trainer and was living what I thought was a conventionally healthy lifestyle, I just continued to grow sicker and sicker.

After reading this book and being introduced to the Law of Attraction and realizing I was in control of my life, I began reading everything I could get my hands on of personal development. Between my alternative health books and my new love for personal development, I spent most of my time reading. It was during this time that I was lead to a naturopath who helped identify part of what was making me so deathly ill. I was infested with parasites and was so completely malnourished because they were eating everything I put into my mouth. After some deep cleansing I was starting to feel much better. Though still sick. I could see light at the end of the tunnel, and with my new thought process I felt as though I could move mountains.

During this time I went up to New York with my family to visit relatives, and while I was up there I had a flash of inspiration. I was going to move to Hawaii and start the life of my dreams. I was born in Hawaii but , left when I was very young, so it had always been a dream of mine to go back. I didn't know anyone there, had no money or job, was still very sick, but I was so filled with faith that I set a date to leave in a few months.

All of sudden things started happening. I found an old client of mine that was willing to let me move in and train him as well as cook all his meals, and in return he would be my transportation to and from a job I found, and pay for my living expenses. I was able to come up with the money for a ticket on the exact date of my deadline. I did this before I even found a place to live! I ended up finding the most magical place on the eastern side of Oahu where I had the mountains in my backyard and the beach across the street. The apartment was amazingly gorgeous with huge glass windows and a wraparound porch, and because it was over a garage, I had the most majestic view you could imagine. My landlord even offered to pick me up from the airport! I found the perfect job easily, and for at least a year I felt as if I could walk on water. Having faith and knowing what you want leads to the most amazing results you can imagine.

Faith is spiritual in nature and just by having faith in yourself and your creations your whole life will change.

Relationships

Your relationships are the most underrated aspect of a person's health. Who you are surrounded with on a daily basis has a huge impact on how you think and feel. It is important to have the people in your life reflect where it is you are trying to go. It is human nature to pick up the qualities that you see each day, and by choosing to associate with those you wish to emulate you naturally start to pick up their qualities and habits.

It's so important to have role models in life. Being able to look to another who you admire gives you a path in which to follow if you want to end up where they did. All teachers begin as students, and a wise man doesn't try and recreate the road to success, but rather follow the path that successful people have already taken.

41

Much less energy is spent, and by putting your attention on learning from others you will naturally develop your own voice and way in time. Everyone is unique and has a unique history. We all have learned different lessons, and everyone has a personalized perception so there is no risk in worrying about becoming a copycat. Learn as much as you can and when the time is right you will naturally be ready to make your own contribution.

Finding your role models is easier than you think. You don't have to know them personally and they don't have to even be alive. You can connect with the best minds in history through books, audiotapes, music, movies and anything that allows you to make a connection and feel their influence in your life.

One of the most important role models in my life is the founder and main teacher for the Institute for Integrative Nutrition, Joshua Rosenthal. He has a calmness and gentleness in his voice and way that naturally puts people at ease. A visionary by nature he took incredible action and created a school that brings to the world the next generation of health practitioners. He saw a world need and filled it. It takes tremendous courage, compassion, and love in your heart to want to help heal the world.

Another vital role model I have is Napoleon Hill. At a young age, Andrew Carnegie (the steel giant) gave him the mission of discovering the laws of success by spending at least 20 years studying and interviewing the greatest minds and most successful people in the world. The result is that millions of people now have a blueprint they can use to achieve any goal. I try to make it a habit to read something he wrote every day. Keeping the laws of success in your mind and drilling them into your subconscious is imperative to reaching any goal you may have in life. One of the most important lessons he continues to teach me every day is nothing in life is ever achieved without a positive mental attitude.

A positive mental attitude is what keeps you going when things look bleak. Being reminded that every adversity has the seed of an equivalent or greater benefit is like having a light in a dark tunnel. Having faith that things will not only get better, but they will get as good as your thoughts allow you to think are just some of the amazing lessons he has taught me.

It is also very important to keep every relationship you have harmonious. Besides the fact that you don't want to attract negativity in your life, the people that you have chosen to be a part of your life are there to help you and you to help them. Listen to others and you will learn so much and save yourself so much time and energy learning the lessons on your own. After all we have so much to do in this lifetime why learn things the hard way and waste valuable time and energy?

Another of the many wonderful things the great Napoleon Hill has taught me is the beauty of having a mastermind alliance. A mastermind alliance can speed up the delivery of a goal because you are increasing the power of thought. The definition of a mastermind alliance is that "The mastermind principle consists of an alliance of two or more people working in harmony for the attainment of a common objective. No two minds ever come together without a third invisible force which may be likened to a "third mind". When a group of individual minds are coordinated and function in harmony, the increased energy created through that alliance becomes available to every member of the group."

When trying to achieve any goal or when simply needing feedback on your plans, having a mastermind alliance is invaluable. No matter how much you know, you are always limited by your own perception. No one ever achieved greatness completely on their own. Support is essential in life and the more support you have the greater power you possess.

It's also very important to be kind to all those who cross your path in life. I believe everyone you come in contact with is for a reason, and at different times and different interactions you may be the teacher or the student. Maybe you are destined to meet someone briefly that confirms a question you have been replaying in your mind, or maybe you were destined to brighten someone's day with a smile or compliment that has a domino effect on their life. You may not know or ever discover all the things in life you influence, but you can rest assured that it is much more than you could ever believe.

Having a strong support system is also necessary for success and peace of mind. All of life is relationships, and you need to have people you can depend on just as much as you need to be depended on. No one ever achieved great success without having support.

I learned firsthand the importance of having a strong support system. When I was approaching the 2 year mark of living in the paradise of Hawaii, I began to lose my way. I still loved Hawaii, had a thriving business, and was working on my physical health, but somewhere along the way I began to let negativity creep into my life. Instead of practicing my philosophies, I felt almost as if they didn't apply to me because of the knowledge I possessed. My health suffered and I had no one to turn to. After all, my family and close friends were on the mainland. I began to grow very lonely and depressed and just wanted to come home. However, when I got back I felt like such a failure I couldn't relax and enjoy the people I missed so badly. My health continued on a downward spiral and if not for the love and support of those closest to me, I am not sure I would have made it through.

Show the people closest to you that you love and care with every interaction you have. You don't know when they will save your life by just being there for you, and you forget how much you are helping theirs by being there for them.

Your mate is one the most important people in your life. Who you choose to be that person is one of the most important decisions you will make. This relationship is vital to keep harmonious. This person is your partner in helping you build the life of your dreams.

It is crucial that there is not only a mutual love, but also a mutual respect and consideration. This person should keep you balanced and make you feel safe and secure. When life gets hard (as it always does at times), you need to be able to rely on them to make you feel better and to shed a new perspective on the situation. Sometimes all you need is a little encouragement, and sometimes it is helpful to see the situation through different eyes. Give and receive love and keep this relationship strong.

Remember that you have a relationship with everything in your life. What you decide to put into to your relationships and in your life, is what you are going to get back.

Physical Activity

The body is the home to your soul, and what you choose to do every day makes a big impact on the comfort level you feel. Did you know that people think of their bodies more than any other subject? The mind-body phenomenon is so powerful that we discover more and more about the incredible link each day. Did you know that your decisions each day on how to treat your body are directly related to how you are treating your brain and emotions? Have you ever wondered why when you live a sedentary existence it is so hard not to have stagnation in your life? Bodies are made to be in motion just as life is meant to progress, and as you increase your physical activity and your entire being gets healthier, you will naturally start to move forward in your life.

The body is made up of cells. The health of each of your cells is the health of your brain, heart, skin, hair, lungs and everything else that is a part of you. To thrive, they need excellent nourishment and a good system of daily detoxification. When waste removal is inhibited and toxins begin to build up in the cells your radiance dims and the ability your cells have to talk to one another is severely impaired. As a result, your reaction times slow, you experience brain fog and your energy diminishes. The body is always in the process of detoxification and the biggest help you can give it is exercise. The more you sweat the more waste is excreted. Exercise stimulates your lymph nodes to dump waste and your lungs to work more efficiently. Your heart grows stronger and your blood becomes cleaner. Remember you want ALL your organs of elimination to work optimally so you can feel your best.

It is also important to remember that you need your muscles and bones to be strengthened as they protect you, hold up your body, and make your day-to-day life much easier. Weight bearing exercises are your best defense against osteoporosis and getting a better body composition. Ever seen a skinny fat person? That happens as the result of lack of muscle of their bodies.

What you don't use you lose. Most people don't realize this, but your muscles and bones are alive. When you don't give them the nourishment from food and stimulation from movement, they atrophy at a very fast rate.

The week after I turned 21 I got in a brutal car accident. I shattered my left femur and humorous (the big bones in my left arm and leg) as well as fractured my pelvis and suffered severe brain trauma, resulting in amnesia and slight brain damage. I had titanium rods placed in both my arm and leg and waited for the bones to grow back around them so I could relearn to walk. The problem was my bones weren't growing back! I now recognize that through my lifestyle I had leeched so many of the minerals in them I was stunting their growth. Not to mention that while I was in my wheelchair, in my depressed state, I was smoking a pack a day, eating a poor diet and the only movement I was attempting was to get from my bed to the wheelchair and back again. I couldn't even wheel myself around because my arm was still in a sling.

This went on for about 6 months and the doctors basically told me that it was unlikely I would walk again. I decided I no longer wanted to be in a world where I was going to be an invalid and not even be able to take a shower without help. I took 2 bottles of sleeping pills and decided I was going to say goodbye to this lifetime and hoped that I was going to a better place. As I lay dying, I called the boyfriend I had gotten in the car accident with and started saying goodbye. I guess he heard a drop or something along those lines because when my side of the connection was gone he knew something was wrong. He called the ambulance and they arrived just in time to save my life.

I woke up in the hospital with even worse brain damage, and the doctors telling my poor mother that they didn't even know if I would speak coherently again. Instead of releasing me, they put me in a state mental hospital. I cannot even describe how horrified I was during my mandatory 2 week stay. When I was released, I decided I was going to fix myself. I learned all I could about the body and how to regenerate physically. Then I started the process of putting myself back together. I

started going to physical therapy and amazed the

therapists so much (who had been told the same things by

the doctors) that they made me a case study. I even

started seeing a neuro-psychiatrist and began to get my

cognitive function back.

As a result of all the exercise, change in diet, and

study, I saw amazing things start to happen in all areas of

my life. I felt better and more grounded than ever before

and was amazed that all processes in my body were

functioning at a higher level. This experience proved to

me, without a shadow of a doubt, how all systems in the

body are connected and when you work to improve one

you are really improving all of them.

When striving to improve your body, one of the

most neglected and important area is your cardiovascular

system. I think people pay less attention to their heart and lungs because they don't see them every day in the mirror, but they need to be shown love as much or more than the rest of you!

The heart is the core of your being and it is also a muscle. It grows or atrophies depending on what you do just like any other muscle. More people die from heart disease than anything else. When you love yourself, you want to protect the muscle that is the center of your being. Aerobic exercise is the best defense against heart disease. A good defense is the best offense. Aerobic exercise can also stimulate the production of serotonin and dopamine, two feel good chemicals. One of the best ways to exercise your cardiovascular system is to jump on a mini-trampoline, also called rebounding. The action of jumping up and down stimulates your lymphatic system to start dumping waste. Your muscles and organs are strengthened and your whole being is revitalized. One of the best things about rebounding is it puts very little strain on your body so you don't have to worry about injury.

It would not be complete to talk about exercise without talking about the benefits of yoga. Yoga is the single most beneficial exercise a person can do. It increases muscle tone and flexibility, detoxifies through breath, and strengthens the mind-body connection. Weight usually falls away when you start practicing yoga because you are naturally more mindful of what you feed yourself. I find that people who practice yoga have a natural grace and ease about them. There is no better feeling than being in tune with your body, and yoga could easily be the quickest way to do that.

All in all, you cannot be truly healthy unless you incorporate some form of movement into your life every day. An easy way to start is to simply walk. Almost anyone can walk no matter what their level of health and everything you do adds up. Start parking farther away from the places you frequent. Make it a habit to be more active during your day by stopping what you are doing every so often and do some squats or simply stretch. EVERYTHING ADDS UP! Life is never all or nothing, but more about the daily habits and practices that you employ. Do things you enjoy like dance or sports. Get outside on a beautiful day and horse around with your kids or play with your dog. Having fun is the ultimate exercise because you tend to forget that's what you're actually doing!

So the goal for exercise - MOVE MORE EVERY DAY.

Career

The ideal career is something you enjoy doing. We want to be spending the hours of the day doing something that moves us. Too many people feel trapped in a job they hate. When you find yourself in that position, it's wise to make a gradual change. You don't want to quit your job and suddenly end up broke without a clue as to what to do. That would only make things worse.

Find something you love that you would do even if you weren't getting paid and figure out a way to get paid to do it! Like everything in life, to succeed at this requires a sound plan of action. When you know in your heart what you are meant to do and can see yourself doing it, it becomes much easier. Just because you don't like where you're at, it's pointless to make a change if you don't have a clear vision of where you are trying to end up. Without a destination you could end up just going around and around from job to job replaying a similar scenario.

The career you choose should reflect your passions in life. Unfortunately, most people dread the place in which they spent most of their waking hours! They walk around uninspired without the excitement that each of us deserves in life.

An easy way to start making a transition is to sit down and start writing out all the things you love to do. Maybe it's to work with children or animals, maybe it's to be in nature, or maybe you want to do something artistic. Next, a good step is to decide whether you want the responsibility of running your own business or if you prefer working for someone else. Both situations have their ups and downs. Some people don't want to have to worry about covering their own insurance or having to set up their own 401K and retirement plan, while for others the dream of being their own boss and having direct control far outweigh the extra work that is required when running your own business.

Another option is deciding you want to simply raise your children. If you are financially able to make that decision that can be one of the most fulfilling jobs there is. Whatever you decide is right for you, do the best job you can and you will reap amazing rewards.

When I was younger, all I knew was that I wanted to make a lot of money. I grew up poor and I vowed I would not end up that way. I was 18 when I entered the world of exotic dancing. Having grown up dancing ballet, modern, tap, jazz and doing gymnastics, this seemed like a wonderful opportunity to do something I love and simultaneously make a lot of money.

For the first couple of years I was unable to see how the environment was affecting me. I may have loved to dance, but I hated everything else that went with it. I couldn't continue to do it without being on drugs or alcohol. Once I could see how badly this was hurting me, I was so used to the money I found it very hard to stop. I would quit for a time, but I always ended up going back. I had a serious conflict in my priorities. It took a complete reorganization of not only my priorities, but my morals and values as well, before it was no longer an option for me.

Realizing my passion lay in health and wellness helped point me in the direction of finding a career that would fulfill me, but I still had to experiment within the field to find work that truly made me happy. Writing allowed me to have a creative outlet while simultaneously making me feel like I was making a contribution to the world.

Finding your niche in your chosen field is like the beginning in a beautiful relationship. As with any relationship, to make it work requires consistent time and effort. Though the rewards for doing work you love is unparalleled.

It's very important when choosing a career that it is in complete harmony with the values you have as a person. You want to be able to give yourself completely with no reservations to whatever you decide to do. Since we are trying to become our ideal person, a good question to ask is, "Is this the career I would choose when I am living my ideal life as my ideal reflection of myself?" If it's not, it's time to sit down and figure out what you do want and create a plan on how to get it. The first steps are always the hardest. Newton's first law of motion is, "A body at rest tends to stay at rest, and a body in motion tends to stay in motion, unless the body is compelled to change its state." If you don't like where you're at, change your state and start moving in the direction you want to go. You will naturally pick up speed as you go along.

Nutrition

If Primary foods are what sets the foundation for your health, then the building blocks you use to create yourself is most definitely your nutrition. There are so many nutritional theories out there it can be very confusing when trying to determine what to feed yourself. Everyone is unique and when you are trying to figure out what nourishes you it is important to remember that your dietary needs should be personalized as well.

That being said there are some core concepts everyone should be aware of. First off it is very important to make all your choices for what you put into your body whole foods. Processed foods are the root of modern disease and it's hard to trust labels because manufacturers sneak damaging ingredients in under different names and the FDA doesn't even make them claim everything if it is under a certain percentage. Did you know you can put no Trans fats on your product as long as it under .5 grams? Pretty scary what our government allows in favor of big business over the general public.

People today do not eat near enough fruits and vegetables! In America, fruits and vegetables only make up 8% of the diet, with half of that coming in the form of french fries and potato chips! Hippocrates, the father of medicine, tells us in plain English, "Let food be thy medicine". No wonder we have an epidemic of sick and obese people. No one is eating their medicine! If health is one of your pursuits in life you MUST eat a wide variety of fruits and vegetables. The RDA is 5 servings but people really should be getting as close to 9 as they can. It's really not that hard, just make half your plate of whatever you are eating vegetables and have fruit for breakfast. The amount of vitamins and minerals you will start taking in will make you feel like a new person. Your body will let out a huge exhale and say thank you.

Michael Pollan said it best when he said "Eat food. Not too much. Mostly plants". If you stick to that regimen, you really can't go wrong. Now when deciding on sides to have with your plants, that's where the individuality comes in. Since we are taking in all this great plant nutrition, it is important for us to allow them to get to work cleaning out the sludge in our bodies without contributing to more of it. So it is important to figure out what your body likes and doesn't. I'm talking about your body and not your taste buds! Most people have food allergies and finding out what yours might be will make a huge difference in your state of well-being. For instance most people can't tolerate gluten and don't know it. Therefore, steady rises in inflammation increase day by day since so many foods have gluten in them. The vast majority of people in the world do not have the enzyme lactase necessary to break down the lactose in dairy and so they create an abundance of mucus in their system that their body has to fight with constantly. Sugar is pretty toxic for everybody, but when you have parasites or an imbalance of good and bad bacteria in your body ALL things that break down into a form of sugar feeds these bad guys and not you. That includes bread, potatoes, fruits, fruit juice, alcohol, rice, cereal, and all forms of dessert.

I can relate to this because after the amount of antibiotics and medication I had due to the car accident, I would up with a very serious imbalance of good and bad bacteria in my own body. I had it for so long, that it changed forms into a yeast/fungus that drilled holes into my intestinal wall and caused a disease known as "leaky gut syndrome". Having a porous intestinal wall allowed microbes and other bad guys to travel throughout my body making me very ill. If I were to consume gluten, an autoimmune reaction would occur and damage my thyroid. The body is a system where everything you do affects your whole body and it all starts with what we put in our mouth. Dr. Mark Hyman has a Functional Medicine wellness center in Massachusetts that I was blessed enough to go to. He helps you to understand that food is information that tells your body what to do. He is a pioneer in the rapidly arising world of Functional Medicine that I believe is our future. Instead of looking at the body as separate parts, the way the western world has always viewed it, they look at the body like a whole and they take out what's bad for it while giving what it needs. Your diet is changed, the bad guys are killed off and your deficiencies are corrected. Soon your body starts to function like it's supposed to and you feel much better!

Now I eat mostly fruits and vegetables with sides of lean protein or a gluten free grain. I find that I do well with minimal amounts of animal protein. Some may do better having animal protein every day, but I strongly encourage you not to make the portion larger than the palm of your hand. You will digest small amounts better and by combining your protein with a significant amount of vegetables, the uric acid and ammonia that are by products of the metabolism of animal protein won't affect you as badly. When shopping for your meats it is important that you go organic whenever possible. Factory farmed animals are given massive amounts of hormones and antibiotics and you have to remember that whatever was injected into them is going into your body to become a part of you.

Raw foods are also very important to have in your diet. When a food is heated to 118 degrees or above, all the enzymes are killed off. You are born with a finite amount of enzymes in your body and the only way to add more is through enzyme supplements and raw food. When food is heated it also kills off about 80% of the vitamins and minerals.

Enzymes are the catalysts for every function that goes on in your body. As you deplete your enzyme reserve, aging occurs. When you eat a significant portion of your diet raw, you guarantee that you keep replenishing your enzyme bank account. Kimberly Snyder writes in her amazing book, The Beauty Detox Diet, that it is a good idea to coat your stomach before meals by eating something raw. This will help make sure you consume a good amount of raw food every day. She also talks about her glowing green smoothie and how consuming it will not only add a bunch of raw goodness, but it is also an excellent way to drop pounds fast. She explains in detail how more energy in the body equals more beauty and has a sound plan to rebalance the body and increase beauty energy.

I think the easiest way to insure you are getting plenty of raw fruits and vegetables is to aim to consume fruit for breakfast and at least one giant salad every day. Personally, I am a huge fan of green juices. By juicing your vegetables, your body spends no additional energy having to break down the fiber and you instantly absorb a bounty of vitamins, minerals, and enzymes. For those who struggle to get their vegetable servings in every day, juicing can be a lifesaver. I love my cucumber-zucchini-celery juice in the morning, and sometimes I throw some ginger in for an additional dose of antioxidants. You can consume massive nutrition in a very short amount of time and I find green juices to be the best source of hydration.

Keeping yourself hydrated is critical since the body is up to 70% water. The most important time to rehydrate is in the morning. Our bodies are still in detox mode and need the water to help flush out toxins. Living with the cycles that your body goes through makes understanding what you should put into your body, and when, much easier.

Cleansing is something your body does all day long and you make it much easier on yourself when you eat in a way that assists the body in doing its job instead of hindering it. You can greatly help your body by properly digesting what you eat so you don't store as much waste. To do this you have to understand how long foods actually take to digest and learn how to eat in combinations that make digestion optimal. This is where food combining comes into play.

Food combining has been used by the natural health community for a long time and I am surprised that it is not well known. My all-time favorite health book, <u>Fit for Life II</u> by Harvey and Marilyn Diamond, goes into detail on the importance of properly combining your food as well as many other important subjects.

Food combining is pretty simple. All foods have a certain length of time they are in the stomach. Fruit is the easiest to digest and takes approximately 30 minutes with melons taking only 20 and bananas 45. If anything else goes into the stomach during this time it holds up digestion and the fruit will sit and ferment in your stomach, acidifying your entire meal. Therefore, it is imperative that you only eat fruit alone and on an empty stomach. The only exception to this rule is the addition of dark leafy greens, making green smoothies an excellent choice for breakfast.

Vegetables combine well with protein and starches, but you should never eat your protein and starches in the same meal. Proteins require an acidic environment in the gut, while starches require an alkaline environment. When they are combined, different digestive enzymes are secreted and they wind up canceling each other out. Nothing digests properly and you wind up with protein that putrefies and starches that ferment, creating a breeding ground for unhealthy bacteria in your intestinal tract. The other problem when eating those foods together is it makes their digestion time increase from 3 hours when eaten alone or with some vegetables, to up to 8 hours when combined! That means you will generally eat again before you have completely digested the meal and because your energy has to switch to digest a new meal, whatever was in the stomach will be stored as waste. As Natalia Rose talks about in her book, The Raw Food Detox Diet, Waste=Weight, and the key to having a slender physique is to eat foods in quick exit combinations.

Living in the real world, I know that it is sometimes impossible for you to combine all your meals perfectly. What happens when your favorite foods are spaghetti and meatballs or tuna sushi rolls? If you MUST miscombine your meal, try to do so at dinner and don't eat anything afterwards. Your body will have all night to go about its work and you can minimize the amount of waste that is stored.

You will be amazed when you start combining your food properly at how much weight will naturally start to fall off. There will also be much less pressure on your veins and arteries without all the gases from fermentation. Try it for a week and see how much better you feel and see how quickly your stomach starts to flatten out!

Another important thing to remember when eating your meals is to SLOW DOWN. Digestion starts in the mouth and you help your body out significantly when you chew your foods well. It takes 20 minutes for your body to realize you're full anyway, so by slowing down you will naturally eat less.

So many people are looking to lose weight and just by eliminating the waste you create by combining your foods properly, slowing down so you know when your full and eating meals with a high nutrient density, you won't have to go on any kind of diet for your weight to naturally stabilize to where your body wants it to be.

Be kind to yourself and feed your body what it needs to thrive. The vast majority of people in America are overfed and undernourished and we are seeing a huge epidemic of disease as a result. Don't let yourself be a statistic. Choose to cherish yourself by making the decision to only put into your temple that which will

cause it to shine.

Becoming Effective

Having all the knowledge in the world will do you no good if you don't apply what you know. Learning the right steps to take is also essential so we don't overwhelm ourselves with trying to do everything. It is important to make sure the changes you are making in your life are done in the right order so you can maximize effectiveness.

Having meaning and purpose in your life is critical to having a healthy outlook. I think the best way to begin to find your purpose is to ask yourself, "What does happiness mean for me?" Being happy is everyone's ultimate goal, after all what's the point in doing anything if you don't wind up feeling fulfilled and satisfied at the end of the day? Finding what brings you joy is the first step in creating a roadmap towards a life you want to live.

When you think of anything in your life and any destination you want to reach, it is important to think 'big picture'. You want your goals and aspirations to be so huge you could never reach them all, thereby you always have something you are striving towards and you are always looking to better yourself. Even if all are met, the journey will create new desires within you so you will never run out of new and exciting adventures. Taking small steps each day in the direction of where you want to end up assures you of enjoying the entire process of manifesting your dreams.

Once you figure out what it is that makes you happy it is important to ask yourself how you can be happy right now. Happiness is not some far off place that you have to travel to. Happiness is letting go of the past and future and being content in the present. The present is the only place we can live anyway. Each moment is precious and it is a wise man that treats each day and encounter as if it could be his last.

A good way to be effective is to practice having control over your state. If you are sad make yourself laugh, even if nothing is funny! Maybe try doing a little dance or turning on a good piece of music. Whatever you can do to change your emotions from negative to positive will be dramatically effective at controlling your life. We are in control of our responses! Events are just events; it's your reaction and interpretation of events that determine how you will feel.

Once you feel you are on the right road to get to where you want to go and have good control over your state then you can start to focus your attention on your actions.

Steven Covey explains the 80/20 rule in his wonderful book, <u>The Seven Habits of Highly Effective</u>

<u>People</u>. This rule shows you that 20% of what you do in life will determine 80% of your results. Understanding the difference between an urgent task and an important task is a vital piece of information that will change your life in itself. An urgent task is something that comes up and needs to be handled right away. An urgent task might be important like calming a screaming baby, but most often they are not, like when the telephone rings. An important task is something that might not be urgent, but will make a big difference in the quality of your life. Exercise is a prime example of an important, but not urgent task. Going back to school or spending time in self-study to further your career may not be urgent, but you will see vast improvements when you make room for these important endeavors.

Spending a portion of each day on issues that are important, but not urgent, will allow you to make the most progress in the shortest amount of time. The more time and effort you spend on these tasks, the greater the rewards.

When you decide to make radical changes in your life, it is best to start off slow. Laying a solid foundation of good habits is much more important than taking on everything in your life at once. This helps you get in the groove and makes change a pleasant experience (an absolute must) and keeps you from burning yourself out.

Look at what changes are going to cause the greatest impact on your life with the littlest effort. Remember your body needs to get warmed up and it's best to start with things that are the easiest for you to control. If you are unhappy in your job, but you are only just beginning to think about other options, it is not wise to make finding a new job your first priority. Just start thinking of other things you may like to do. Keep it light and just start putting it out there to the world and your subconscious to keep your eyes and ears open for opportunities.

One thing you are 100% in control of is your diet. What you order off a menu or buy at the grocery store is completely up to you. When people make healthy nutrition choices it affects everything. Eating healthier may not change the world, but it will make your world a much nicer place to be. It's so much easier to think positive when your body is feeling good and your body is just not going to feel its best when running off of subpar fuel. Sugar and bad fats may spike serotonin briefly but the long term consequences and the toll it takes on your body and mind is much more substantial to your overall happiness in life.

When changing your diet, it is best to start with the things that will give you the best results without drastically altering your way of life. This is best achieved by increasing the amount of fruits and vegetables in your diet while taking out the worst things for your body. White flour and white sugar are the worst things for your body to be running off of. They result in major insulin spikes followed by crashes causing you to crave more of them and all day long and your body gets put on this rollercoaster of highs and lows. Sounds awful, doesn't it? Unfortunately, more and more people are doing this all day every day until their bodies start to break down. Your body has to pump out massive amounts of insulin to help lower the sugar spikes. The more sugar you put into your body, the more insulin is needed. This is causing so many people to develop Type II diabetes. Show love and respect for your body by not continually putting poison in it.

Physical activity is something you also want to gradually build up. As you do, you will find yourself with more energy and clearer thinking which will result in your becoming much more effective. Without proper physical activity your body is just not going to run as well. When your physical body doesn't run optimally, can you really expect your mind to? How can you be effective in your life when your mind and body aren't working efficiently?

Another activity that most people do not prioritize is their sleeping habits. Sleep is when the body restores its energy and heals its wounds. Sleep is the only time many of us are not spending most of our energy digesting food and this frees up energy in the body to do all its repair work. We need this down time! As you get older you will feel the effects of not getting enough sleep much more profoundly. You will wind up tired and cranky when you lack sufficient sleep. The recommended

amount of sleep a night is 7-8 hours, but like everything,

people differ on the amounts they need and it is important

to listen to the body.

Constant Education

The habit of constantly educating yourself is one of the most powerful ways to get where you want to go in life. While some people may be lucky and are born with innate talents, talent will only get you so far. In order to truly become skilled at anything you must practice hard work, dedication, discipline, and above all consistent learning. Most people think their education ends with their formal schooling, but really that should be the start if you really want to achieve great success in your field. New information is constantly coming to the surface and without the practice of constantly seeking more knowledge there is little doubt you will fall behind.

When educating yourself, it is important to remember that like everything else there are numerous ways to go about doing it. There are traditional schools, online education, books, audiotapes, mentoring programs, you can always find a way to learn that fits your schedule and preferred method of learning. The important thing is that you consistently grow and expand your knowledge. Proactively taking charge of your life and the practice of self-study go hand in hand. Remember, leaders are readers! If you want to be a leader in your chosen field this is a step you CANNOT skip.

The Key to Success

The key to success in any undertaking and in life itself is your mindset. The beginning of this book helps you develop a mindset in order to know what you want and to get it. I want to close by explaining the two main types of mindsets and how they will affect not only all your outcomes, but also your happiness while going through life.

The first mindset I want to talk about is the fixed mindset. A fixed mindset believes that your intelligence, health, skill set, and basic personality is all predetermined at birth. You already have all the skills you're going to have in life, so it becomes necessary to protect yourself and your confidence by doing what you're naturally good at, forsaking all chances to grow and develop. With this backwards thinking, you take so much pleasure out of life because you don't see all your past attempts where you may have failed as learning opportunities on your way to success. Someone with the fixed mindset doesn't get excited by challenges and rarely gets to experience all that life has to offer. Don't let yourself fall prey to the fixed mindset which doesn't allow you to grow and change. We are not our past experiences, our bodies, or even our future. We are spiritual beings having a physical experience and we should appreciate every moment and embrace all challenges as opportunities to refine our skills and better ourselves.

The flip side to the fixed mindset is the growth mindset. With the growth mindset firmly in place there really is no limit to what you can accomplish. Even when you may be particularly lacking in skill at something, you know that with time and effort all things are attainable.

Having the belief that you are always evolving and becoming better puts you in the right frame of mind for success. A lack of ability motivates you to work harder or smarter. If you still don't achieve results, you don't put yourself down; instead you realize that you may need to change your approach. Someone with a growth mindset doesn't recognize defeat as anything more than a temporary setback in which you have ability to learn what doesn't work and adjust yourself accordingly. People with a growth mindset rarely stay at the bottom for long because they appreciate and take advantage of each opportunity to better themselves. They learn from their mistakes and they don't beat themselves up. Having this mindset also allows your confidence to grow and your experience of life to be much more enjoyable.

Time passes for us all and as we experience the different stages in life a growth mindset is essential. Life is a never ending classroom and it is important to learn as much as you can during each phase so that you don't have to repeat the same lessons. When you choose to learn and grow from your trials and tribulations this allows those lessons to leave your life and make room for the next ones that are to come. When you don't take the time to learn, you will always wind up in a similar situation or circumstance that causes you to repeat the lesson. Some people go through life repeating the same "grade" over and over again. This happened to me for years; I would make minor variations of the same scenario and wondered why I wasn't getting drastically different results. Save yourself the time and trouble and learn and grow from all your experiences so you can move on and experience more of what life has to offer. Remember, you will always have life lessons but learning to embrace them is how you achieve a growth mindset.

For more extensive information on the fixed mindset and the growth mindset please check out Mindset, by Carol S. Dweck, PH. D

Living Life

We all want to have full, enriching, happy lives. Sometimes we spend so much time trying to achieve, that we don't take the time to enjoy the process of living. Getting caught up in unimportant, temporary, superficial aspects can pave the way to a life filled with stress, depression, and anxiety. Recognize that you are already a success and that whatever you choose to do to better yourself is just going to help make the journey that much more enjoyable. Having a healthy body, a creative and fulfilling career, and nurturing relationships are all just tools to elevate your satisfaction in life. Life is temporary and it goes by so fast, don't waste a second of it. Learn to live without regret and be sure to cherish yourself along the way.

Letter From

a Client

Letter from a client . . .

A colleague at work told me about her daughter Shana Perkins over the years we have worked together. I found myself inspired by what little I knew of her life story. I heard how she was able to transform her health and body from adverse circumstances. So, when I was provided the opportunity for Shana's coaching for my fitness and weight loss I jumped on it. Here is my story:

I have always been fairly active but that activity has gone in spurts. In between those spurts I gained weight and got more and more out of shape. When I was in my teens and early 20's I was an avid long distance runner and extremely fit. There was a period of time that I ran 15 miles a day at a 7 minute pace, could run 1 mile in 5 minutes and 5 miles in 30 minutes. I could climb up a 50 foot rope and back down just using my arms. Then education, marriage, children, work and life all happened which pulled me more and more away from regular activity. The problem is that things downgrade so gradually that you don't notice. But, like the boiling frog experiment where it doesn't realize it's in boiling water until it's too late, my weight went up and my fitness went down and I, like the frog, I did not fully realize what was happening to me.

When I turned 40 I had regained a fairly high level of fitness for that age. I could run 5 miles fairly easily and do 24 strict form pull ups. That was a great 'spurt' but the benefits were predominantly cosmetic in nature. This past year as I turned 49 I was far from that level and realized that something needed to happen. I had regressed to a dangerous level, the type that my doctors were starting to worry about. Just 2 years ago my doctor told me I had metabolic syndrome. That's a nice way of letting you know your fat. My belly measured 45 inches. My 42 inch waist pants were tight on me. My weight was up to 249 pounds and I had to take medication for cholesterol and high blood pressure. I had to sleep with a CPAP device for sleep apnea and literally could not see my feet. I also suffered from depression which meant it was hard to care about anything and get motivated to do anything and I ate to reduce stress. I loathed life in general.

If I needed someone in my life to help me it was then. This is when my 19 year old cousin was transferred to Ft. Bragg about an hour away from my home. He was my first stage. My cousin due to his age and due to the high conditioning of the army special forces was in extremely good shape. He took interest in me his elder cousin over twice his age and inspired me to be serious about working out again. Through his inspiration and help I began run/walking and doing body weight exercises (pullups, pushups, squats). I also used suspension strap training as well.

This allowed me to reduce my weight to 234 pounds and to stop taking my blood pressure and cholesterol medications. Knowing that my 50th birthday was coming up in July I had the fortune of having Shana Perkins come into my life in March. This was perfect timing as my cousin was in Afghanistan and his advice was mainly from an exercise standpoint. My cousin brought me close to where I was at age 40 but I was not progressing further. Shana started slow with me and asked me to do some things that caused me to give pause so she would often say, "David, humor me and try this for a week". The first week I dropped 7 pounds! Each week or two we would tweak things with my diet and/or exercise. It was an abrupt lifestyle change and was hard at first but I was motivated. Shana also talked to me about my life and what stressors I faced and how I handled them. She indeed took a whole life approach and went far beyond what a normal trainer would do. In fact, diet and exercise were only about half of what we talked about. She indeed took me to levels that I thought would be impossible-especially with my age. I have gained a new respect for what the human body can do, how it can be pushed and how it can respond and reward you when you give it good nutrition and put it to hard work and teach it to relax.

My goal now physically is to have visible abs and almost there. I have 2-pack abs. The other 4 cans of beer are still hiding. My mother cannot stop showing recent pictures of me to everyone. My wife can't keep her hands off me- this is new and welcomed! Part of my motivation early in this process was due to the fact that I turned 50 but another part now is that I want to help others. If I can do this anyone can! I really mean that too, by the way. I see too many colleagues, family and friends that approach this milestone of mid-life overweight, out of shape and suffering various health problems as a result- like I did. That is not and should not be considered normal and part of being 50! So, I seriously started this journey back in March of this year with the help of Shana.

Prior to this latest life change program I took a bodybuilder approach to fitness. That's what most personal trainers and gyms promote one to do and I followed suit like a starry eyed cult member. High amounts of protein, high calories with little emphasis on cardio work and no emphasis on how many toxins or 'hard to digest' things I was eating. Let me tell you; generally this approach is not healthy and can actually be even harmful to your body. You may look great but you are NOT healthy. I often wondered why the typical body builder was hard pressed to run over 2 miles. A lot of this philosophy has now been turned upside down for me and I'm thankful.

My current exercise routine is very simple; Every morning I spend 15 minutes on a rebounder. The benefits of rebounding deserve their own book. One that I will mention is that it has kept my skin tight despite all the weight loss. I may also do a quick short run or a brisk long walk on my non running days. 3 evenings I do weight bearing strength work;

pushups, pullups, squats, clean and press, crunches, etc. I add finisher exercises occasionally using my TRX. The other 4 days I do cardio- usually in the evening but, I'm trying to do more in the mornings- especially during the Summer. I do a mixture of interval training (run/walk) or endurance runs. Outside of this regimen I make sure I have as many active outings as I can (ex; hiking) every week. I also do Yoga and stretch a lot to work on my flexibility- one can never do enough of that.

My diet is also very radical to how it has been in the past. Know that you will be teased, even ridiculed about what you eat. Do not let that impede your resolve. Let your results speak for themselves; I buy only organic when possible. Here is an example; breakfast; a spinach and frozen banana smoothie with flax seeds added; AM snack; 10 soaked almonds; Lunch; mixed color baby greens with red salmon, flax powder, hemp protein powder and olive oil; PM snack; kale and avocado; Dinner; cooked green beans, greens with olive oil and hemp protein powder and baked fish or chicken.

My total calories range from 1,250-1,500. This represents approximately a 1,000 calorie per day deficit of what my normal metabolism would burn if I did no exercise. Thus, on average, I'm burning 1-2 pounds of fat a week. On cardio days I have more calories to compensate for the activity. Note; that I have no grains (except for occasional Quinoa or Millet instead of animal protein), no sugar (except for some AM fruit), no alcohol and no starches. Do I feel deprived? NO! This comes from someone who was formally trained as a chef and knows how to eat big! Every 1-2 months I take a 1-3 day break to confuse my metabolism (beer, dessert, pizza, etc). I don't binge during this but eat and drink 'normal' levels and eat and drink what most people would call 'normal'. This carb cycling/metabolism shocking really works and takes the edge off of things being mundane. The funny thing is that I miss my fitness diet when I'm going through one of these breaks! It's all about habit. We crave for what we are used to. The supplements I take are: multivitamins, fish oil, magnesium citrate, Vitamin D3, Calcium Citrate, Probiotics, and B12.

After being on this program for just over 5 months I weigh 204 pounds, I loosely wear 34 inch waist pants and I can report that my energy level is through the roof. I no longer have sleep apnea. I currently look good but still don't yet have 6-pack abs. Starting with a body fat percentage of over 30% I have brought it down to 13%. This may be the lowest it has been since my teenage years. My skin looks 100% better. My libido is like I was 18 years old. No, it's actually better. My BP is averaging 112/70. My resting heart rate is 55. My cholesterol is 130. My ability to concentrate has improved. I can run 3 miles and carry a conversation while doing so. I can do 14 strict form pull ups and 60 pushups without stopping. My strength and endurance continue to rIse while my fat levels continue to drop. Everything, and I mean everything, in my life is getting better and better.

There are a few people in this world who have an angel come into their life. Shana is that angel for me. When I think about how much she has helped me it causes me to cry in gratitude. I'm not a crier so this is a big deal. When we overcome obstacles in our lives I believe that we have both an opportunity and a responsibility to share that with others who want to and need to overcome the same things. The beautiful thing about it is that at this point in your life people will listen and follow you because you practice what you preach. Seeing others imitate you and ask you for advice and make changes in their lives is actually much more rewarding than the good changes you have made for yourself.

One of the numerous benefits to this life change is that it has taught me to listen to my body. It is like having a perfect personal trainer built right inside you. There are times when I need to eat more or less, exercise more or less or rest more or less. I used to ignore signals and paid for it with injuries, burnout and performance drops.

Another benefit of this life change is that you learn to be patient with yourself. Progress is not always linear but your commitment and your motivation must be insatiable. No matter how undisciplined you may be in life you will always do what it takes to avoid pain. When the pain of change exceeds the pain of the 'status quo' you will then change. When you see results as a reward from your sacrifice then that sacrifice no longer is viewed as sacrifice at all. Your thinking will change and the way you look at things, indeed your philosophy will change as well. Suddenly, that beer or that piece of pie is thought of and viewed entirely differently than before you begin this journey. You may start a run and after one minute feel like you can't continue. But, a new voice from within speaks to you and you realize that it is a mental game during your run and suddenly you 'feel' like running, in fact faster and further than your original plan.

I hope that my story can provide you with a glimpse of the transformation that you can make starting today. Like me, you can go to the dentist and 6 months later on your next checkup the dentist will not recognize who you are. Like me, you can have co-workers, without any coaxing start to imitate what you do and later tell you how inspired they are from your example. It starts with one decision and taking things one day at a time.

David

About the Author

Shana Perkins is a certified holistic health counselor and certified personal trainer. She is a graduate of the Institute for Integrative Nutrition and is accredited by the American Association of Drugless Practitioners. Her passion for total wellness was borne out of her own personal health challenges. She is now committed to helping others achieve total health and wellness and understanding their own bio-individuality.